Naoto Nakagawa

Improving habitual reading of clinical literature in Japan

Naoto Nakagawa

Improving habitual reading of clinical literature in Japan

Pharmacy students and current pharmacists

LAP LAMBERT Academic Publishing

Impressum / Imprint

Bibliografische Information der Deutschen Nationalbibliothek: Die Deutsche Nationalbibliothek verzeichnet diese Publikation in der Deutschen Nationalbibliografie; detaillierte bibliografische Daten sind im Internet über http://dnb.d-nb.de abrufbar.
Alle in diesem Buch genannten Marken und Produktnamen unterliegen warenzeichen-, marken- oder patentrechtlichem Schutz bzw. sind Warenzeichen oder eingetragene Warenzeichen der jeweiligen Inhaber. Die Wiedergabe von Marken, Produktnamen, Gebrauchsnamen, Handelsnamen, Warenbezeichnungen u.s.w. in diesem Werk berechtigt auch ohne besondere Kennzeichnung nicht zu der Annahme, dass solche Namen im Sinne der Warenzeichen- und Markenschutzgesetzgebung als frei zu betrachten wären und daher von jedermann benutzt werden dürften.

Bibliographic information published by the Deutsche Nationalbibliothek: The Deutsche Nationalbibliothek lists this publication in the Deutsche Nationalbibliografie; detailed bibliographic data are available in the Internet at http://dnb.d-nb.de.
Any brand names and product names mentioned in this book are subject to trademark, brand or patent protection and are trademarks or registered trademarks of their respective holders. The use of brand names, product names, common names, trade names, product descriptions etc. even without a particular marking in this work is in no way to be construed to mean that such names may be regarded as unrestricted in respect of trademark and brand protection legislation and could thus be used by anyone.

Coverbild / Cover image: www.ingimage.com

Verlag / Publisher:
LAP LAMBERT Academic Publishing
ist ein Imprint der / is a trademark of
OmniScriptum GmbH & Co. KG
Heinrich-Böcking-Str. 6-8, 66121 Saarbrücken, Deutschland / Germany
Email: info@lap-publishing.com

Herstellung: siehe letzte Seite /
Printed at: see last page
ISBN: 978-3-659-80213-3

Improving habitual reading of pharmacy related clinical literature in Japan

Naoto Nakagawa

To my dear wife, Ikuko,

And to my lovely kids, Aoi and Koh

Naoto Nakagawa

CONTENTS

INTRODUCTION

I studied abroad at Nova Southeastern University College of Pharmacy in Florida, United States of America (USA) in 2008. My goal was to determine differences between Japanese and American pharmacy education. After graduation, I reached the conclusion that Japanese pharmacists (myself included) do not habitually read pharmacy related clinical literature. That is a problem with Japanese pharmacy education. On the other hand, American pharmacy students study drug literature evaluation in class (Phillips *et al.*, 2012) and participate in journal clubs. This is an educational group meeting in which members critically discuss new clinical literature and evaluate possible clinical applications of the clinical literature.(Kirchhoff and Beck, 1995) Additionally, preceptors in advanced pharmacy practice experiences (APPE) often assign the journal club to pharmacy interns.(Arif *et al.*, 2012) Therefore, American pharmacy students habitually read clinical literature prior to graduation.

I have felt since graduation that this is one of the reasons

Japanese pharmacy education lags behind American. Almost all Japanese pharmacists have probably been unaware of this. It is my responsibility to show the difference between Japan and the USA and fill the gap between them.

I will discuss a comparative survey of pharmacists' perceptions of clinical literature accessibility between Japan and the USA. I then describe my recommendations to fill the gap between Japan and the USA. These include an evidence-based medicine workshop to increase Japanese pharmacy students' awareness of the importance of reading current clinical literature and using journal clubs to improve medical terminology and critical reading skills. This research verified outcomes in the Department of Pharmaceutical Sciences at Tohoku University Hospital.

1. Comparative Survey of Pharmacists' Perceptions of Clinical Literature Accessibility between Japan and the USA

1.1   Background

American pharmacy students learn how to critically read

clinical literature in classed on drug literature evaluation; APPE preceptors regularly assign journal clubs (group activities in which pharmacy students make an oral presentation critiquing clinical literature) to pharmacy students. On the other hand, in Japan, although pharmacy students utilize fundamental academic literature when they do basic research, they rarely learn how to read academic or clinical literature in class. In addition, the Japanese Pharmaceutical Education Model Core Curriculum (MCC) (http://www.pharm.or.jp/eng/curriculum.html) was revised in 2015 to include practice of evidence-based medicine (EBM), biostatistics, and clinical research design/analysis in the curriculum. However, conventional pharmaceutical education has not emphasized critically reading clinical literature.

1.2 Objectives

To clarify the problems of drug information education in Japan, a comparative survey of pharmacists' perceptions of clinical literature accessibility between Japan and the USA was performed.

1.3 Methods

1.3.1 Questionnaire

The questionnaire is shown in Figure 1. It comprises two sections. Section 1 includes questions on respondents' backgrounds; Section 2 included questions on habitually reading clinical literature. A Japanese version was also created. Google Drive (http://www.google.co.jp) was utilized to create a web questionnaire for American pharmacists in Florida.

1.3.2 Respondent lists

Questionnaires for Japanese pharmacists were sent to those in Miyagi prefecture. Pharmacists in Miyagi prefecture were selected from the website of the Miyagi prefecture government (http://www.pref.miyagi.jp/).

Email addresses for American pharmacists in Florida were retrieved from the website of the Florida Board of Pharmacy (http://floridaspharmacy.gov/). Mailing lists were made based on this information.

1.3.3 Questionnaire distribution

Japanese questionnaires were mailed to pharmacists in Miyagi. An envelope contained an invitation letter, a questionnaire, and a stamped return envelope. A URL of the web questionnaire was emailed to pharmacists in Florida with the title "International Pharmacy Education Research."

1.3.4 Ethical considerations

The ethics committee of Tohoku University School of Medicine, Japan and the institutional review board of Nova Southeastern University College of Pharmacy, USA approved this study. Participation in the questionnaire surveys indicated provision of informed consent.

1.4   Results

Questionnaires were mailed to 1,997 pharmacists in Miyagi and 605 pharmacists responded to questionnaires. URLs were emailed to 18,744 pharmacists in Florida and 171 pharmacists responded to the web questionnaires. Response rate in Miyagi and Florida was 30.3% and 0.91%, respectively. As the responses from the pharmacists in Florida were very low, statistical analysis was not performed.

Backgrounds of all pharmacists were shown in Figure 2. The highest percentage (22.0%) of pharmacists in Miyagi had 1–5 years of pharmacist experience. As pharmacist experience increased, percentages decreased less. However, the highest percentage (27.4%) of pharmacists in Florida had over 30 years of experience.

Of pharmacists, 14.7% in Miyagi (n = 597) and 71.9% (n = 167) in Florida responded that they HABITUALLY read pharmacy related clinical literature (Figure 3). More pharmacists (81.1% of 594 in Miyagi and 92.8% of 167 in Florida) responded that pharmacists need to read clinical literature as part of their regular professional obligations (Figure 4). Of pharmacists who habitually read clinical literature (n = 88 in Miyagi, n = 120 in Florida), frequency was questioned; 34.1% of pharmacists in Miyagi responded monthly and 29.9% of pharmacists in Florida responded more than five times monthly (Figure 5). Similarly, 58.0% of pharmacists in Miyagi and 59.1% of pharmacists in Florida responded "for myself education" as the reason for habitual reading, while 44.3% of pharmacists in Miyagi and 39.6% of pharmacists in Florida did it because it was "necessary in practice" (Figure 5). On the other hand, pharmacists who do not habitually read clinical literature (n = 654 in Miyagi, n = 48 in Florida) were asked why they did not do so; 41.6% of pharmacists in Miyagi and 47.9% of pharmacists in Florida responded "I have no time to read clinical literature" (Figure 6).

Figure 7 shows the results of participants' responses rating their ability to critique/analyze clinical literature (1: Accept it as written/do not critique, 7: Thoroughly critique/analyze) and the extent to which they learned how to critically read clinical literature in pharmacy school (1: Not at all, 7: Yes). Medians of the former in Miyagi and Florida were "2" and "4," respectively (n = 591 in Miyagi, n = 168 in Florida). Medians of the latter in Miyagi and Florida were "1" and "5," respectively (n = 590 in Miyagi, n = 170 in Florida).

Figure 8 shows the extent to which pharmacists apply the information obtained from clinical literature to their daily responsibilities (1: Rarely/Never, 7: Frequently). Medians in Miyagi and Florida were "2" and "5," respectively (n = 573 in Miyagi, n = 170 in Florida).

Figure 9 shows whether pharmacists have access to any clinical studies in their current work environment (1: Not at all, 7: Yes). Medians in Miyagi and Florida were "3" and "5," respectively (n = 573 in Miyagi, n = 170 in Florida).

1.5 Discussion

This study clarified that pharmacists in Florida habitually read clinical literature whereas those in Miyagi did not (Figure 3). Most pharmacists in Florida read clinical literature more than five times per month whereas most pharmacists in Miyagi read clinical literature once a month (Figure 5). Thus, pharmacists in Florida read clinical literature more often than those in Miyagi. Pharmacists in both Miyagi and Florida recognized the necessity of reading clinical literature. Pharmacists in Florida often applied the information obtained from clinical literature to daily practice whereas pharmacists in Miyagi did not (Figure 8). Thus, American pharmacists habitually read clinical literature and applied the information in practice. However, since Japanese pharmacists do not habitually read clinical literature, they did not utilize the information from clinical literature in practice.

Here, the reason why Japanese pharmacists did not habitually read clinical literature is discussed. Most pharmacists in Florida spent time learning how to critically read clinical literature whereas most pharmacists in Miyagi did not (Figure 7). That is why pharmacists in Florida were able to critically read clinical literature whereas those in Miyagi were not. Therefore, since lectures or in-class exercises regarding drug literature evaluation are not provided in Japanese pharmacy schools, pharmacists who habitually read clinical literature are not educated. Figure 2 shows that many pharmacists in Florida whose pharmacist experience was more than 30 years responded to web questionnaires. In the USA, it seems that lectures/exercises regarding article searching started in pharmacy schools in the 1980s (Ikeda and Schwartz, 1992). Experienced pharmacists habitually read clinical literature because drug literature evaluation at pharmacy schools in the USA has been taught for a long time.

There was somewhat of a difference between Miyagi and Florida regarding the question of access to clinical studies in the current work environment. Medians in Miyagi and Florida were "3" and "5," respectively (Figure 9), showing it is necessary to improve work environments for Japanese pharmacists to be able to access clinical literature easily. The difference of access to any clinical literature between Miyagi and Florida affects habitually reading clinical literature. On the other hand, the reason pharmacists do not habitually read clinical literature is that they have no time to do so in both Miyagi and Florida, suggesting that it is necessary to improve work environments for pharmacists in both areas (Figure 6).

This study did have some limitations. First, the response rate from pharmacists in Florida was very low. Because of that, the internal validity of accessibility of clinical literature for pharmacists in Florida was not guaranteed. Second, it is possible that responding pharmacists in Florida tended to be interested in clinical literature. However, as far as I know, this is the first study to discuss accessibility of clinical literature between two nations. Therefore, these data are valuable to improve pharmacy education in Japan.

The MCC was revised in 2015 to include "critically reading clinical literature," specifically, a basic concept of EBM. The number of pharmacy students who take this curriculum will increase in the future and the quality of pharmacy practice will be improved. On the other hand, there is an issue with how current pharmacists learn to critically read clinical literature. Therefore, approaches that teach Japanese pharmacists to critically read clinical literature and then apply the clinical literature information in practice would be necessary.

In conclusion, to clarify problems in drug information education in Japan, a comparative survey of pharmacists' perceptions of clinical literature accessibility between Japan and the USA was performed. As a result, Japanese pharmacists did not sufficiently apply information from the clinical literature in practice because conventional pharmacy education in Japan did not provide lectures/exercises to pharmacy students on how to critically read clinical literature.

2. Japanese pharmacy education for students -Effects of an Evidence-Based Medicine Workshop on Japanese Pharmacy Students' Awareness Regarding the Importance of Reading Current Clinical Literature-

2.1 Background

EBM is well known around the world. Drug literature evaluation courses are taught as in-class activities at almost every college or school of pharmacy in USA. (Wang *et al.*, 2006; Timpe *et al.*, 2006) Journal clubs have been so popular that both pharmacists and pharmacy students alike are able to easily access and critically read clinical literature.(Kleinpell, 2002; Kirchhoff and Beck, 1995) On the other hand, although the MCC in Japan includes an EBM category, it has not provided guidance on how to critically read clinical literature; thus, pharmacy students in Japan do not seem to have critical reading skills for clinical literature. Therefore, some activities are necessary to enhance pharmacy students' skills and awareness of the importance of reading current clinical literature.

Bookstarver et al. reported that EBM courses improve student APPE performance (Bookstaver *et al.*, 2011) in the USA. In this report, we chose to adopt a small class size (5 –6 students) because a small group style is considered one of the most effective instruction methods.

In addition, the Kawakita Jiro (KJ) Method, known as an effective problem-solving technique, has often been utilized in the decision-making process in Japan (Scupin, 1997). Briefly, the KJ method involves the following four essential procedures: 1) label-making (using brainstorming); 2) label- grouping; 3) chart-making; and 4) written or verbal explanations. This method can promote a deeper understanding of problems and exposure to new viewpoints from other students. We considered that an activity involving the KJ Method might help facilitate student understanding of pharmacy-related topics.

2.2 Objectives

To enhance student awareness of the importance of reading clinical literature regularly, we developed an EBM workshop for students. We evaluated its effectiveness using questionnaire surveys administered both before and after the EBM workshop.

2.3 Methods

2.3.1 Orientation

Before the study began, an orientation informed pharmacy students of optional programs given at the beginning of pharmacy practice experiences. During the orientation, students were provided with an outline of the EBM workshop, which included a role-play scenario, required readings, and a suggested reading (Figure 10).

2.3.2 Role-play scenario

Researching a physician's drug information (DI) question is included in pharmacy practice experiences for fifth grade pharmacy students at Tohoku University Hospital; therefore, a role-play scenario involving a conversation between a physician, a ward pharmacist, and a DI pharmacist was created. Briefly, the patient being discussed was a 55-year-old female inpatient with congestive heart failure (New York Heart Association functional classification III) and diabetes. Her left ventricular ejection fraction was 40% two months previously; then, after developing shortness of breath, it decreased to 35% three days previously. The cardiologist considering her treatment asked the ward pharmacist a question (Figure 11).

2.3.3 Required and suggested readings

The pharmacy students were assigned two required readings regarding the clinical literature on valsartan (Cohn and Tognoni, 2001) and candesartan (McMurray et al., 2003) for the role-play. A therapeutic guideline created by the Japanese Circulation Society for patients with chronic heart failure in Japan was also assigned as a suggested reading (The Japanese Circulation Society; http://www.jcirc.or.jp/guideline/pdf/JCS2010_matsuzaki_h.pdf).

These materials were given to the pharmacy students during orientation before the EBM workshop. Based on these readings, the students had to make a decision during the role-play about which drug was better for the patient.

2.3.4 EBM workshop

The EBM workshop was part of a one-day workshop and an elective option in pharmacy practice experiences at Tohoku University Hospital. The EBM workshop consisted of two domains. The first domain involved student presentations of their opinions on critically reading clinical literature. Student presentations were based on required reading; a lecture by a preceptor was given to the students regarding how to read critically in a small group (5–6 students). The other domain used the KJ method (Figure 12) to answer the following two questions: (1) "Is it possible to compare the clinical efficacy of valsartan and candesartan using package inserts and interview forms?" and (2) "How can current evidence be obtained for questions arising or changes occurring after the therapeutic guidelines have been published?"

2.3.5 Evaluation of the EBM workshop using questionnaires

To evaluate the EBM workshop effectiveness, we created questionnaires to administer both before and after participation. The pre-workshop questionnaire was designed to confirm the students' background knowledge of and readiness to read clinical literature. The post-workshop questionnaire was almost the same as the pre-workshop questionnaire, but designed to assess changes in student readiness. Both questionnaires asked students to indicate their level of agreement with statements regarding clinical literature on a seven-point Likert scale (1: strongly disagree, 7: strongly agree; Figures 13A and 13B).

2.3.6 Pre- and post-workshop EBM test

Identical 15-question tests (Figure 14) were administered to the students before and after the workshop to assess their baseline EBM knowledge and to evaluate what they had learned, respectively.

2.3.7 Evaluation of the EBM workshop in optional programs

Pharmacy students in several optional programs evaluated the understanding, satisfaction, and necessity of the EBM workshop at the end of pharmacy practice experiences. This evaluation used a five-point Likert scale (1: not understandable at all, unsatisfying, not necessary at all; 5: completely understandable, very satisfying, extremely necessary).

2.3.8 Statistical analysis

The Wilcoxon signed-rank test was used to determine statistically significant differences between the pre- and the post-workshop questionnaires. The paired Student's t test was used to determine statistically significant differences between the pre- and post-tests. P values less than 0.05 indicated statistical significance.

2.3.9 Ethical considerations

The Tohoku University School of Medicine ethics committee approved this study (No. 2013-1-050). The study purpose was explained to the pharmacy students during orientation for pharmacy practice experiences; participation in the questionnaire surveys indicated provision of informed consent.

2.4 Results

A total of 37 pharmacy students participated in the EBM workshop and 5–6 students per activity attended the small group discussions. The EBM workshop was held eight times between May 2013 and November 2013. Of 37 pharmacy students, 17 students participated in the EBM workshop in the first term of the long pharmacy practice experience and 20 students in the second term.

Partial results of the pre-workshop questionnaire, as well as comparison of student responses between the pre- and post-workshop questionnaires, are shown in Table 1. We found that 57% of the pharmacy students had previously read clinical literature, but 81% had not learned how to read critically.

The results of the EBM workshop evaluations by pharmacy students are shown in Figure 15. Ten students considered the EBM workshop to be mostly understandable and 17 students considered it to be completely understandable. Five students considered the workshop satisfying and 22 students considered it very satisfying. Two students considered the workshop somewhat necessary and 25 considered it extremely necessary.

2.5 Discussion

Although over 50% of the pharmacy students had previously read clinical literature, a majority had not learned how to read such literature critically, suggesting that most pharmacy students do not read clinical literature correctly. Therefore, the EBM workshop is one of the best opportunities to gain awareness of this inability. This suggests that new information from clinical literature would be applied to pharmacy practice when these students become pharmacists in the future. The pre-workshop questionnaire made it clear that most pharmacy students believe that pharmacists should read clinical literature regularly. Furthermore, student awareness of this point significantly increased on the post-workshop questionnaire, suggesting the effectiveness of the EBM workshop. Therefore, it is expected that pharmacy students who participate in EBM workshops, such as those described in the present study, will read clinical literature critically and correctly and apply new information to pharmacy practice in the future. In addition, although scores regarding student confidence in their ability to read clinical literature were low, they significantly increased from 1.81 ± 0.15 before the workshop to 3.92 ± 0.18 after the workshop; however, the post-workshop scores remained under four, indicating an ongoing low level of student confidence. In addition, although scores regarding discussions with physicians and nurses were low, they significantly increased from 2.49 ± 0.22 before to 3.86 ± 0.21 after the workshop; however, these scores also remained low (under four). These results suggest that our EBM workshop needs to be revised in order to significantly increase these scores. For example, one possibility would be to repeat EBM workshops twice or three times in pharmacy practice experiences. Repeated training on clinical decision making based on clinical literature could also be of benefit.

Scores on the EBM pre-test were high (Table 1), indicating that Japanese pharmacy students already understood the EBM concept. Scores on the EBM post-test were slightly higher, but significant, after the EBM workshop, suggesting that it was useful to summarize pharmacy students' EBM knowledge.

A majority of the pharmacy students considered the EBM

workshop to be understandable, satisfying, and necessary (Figure 6). In particular, necessity was the aspect most highly valued by the pharmacy students, suggesting that they were aware that reading clinical literature is necessary for pharmacists. In other words, if the revised MCC includes teaching how to read clinical literature critically, future students will understand the necessity of and appropriate methods for reading clinical literature correctly. Moreover, as these students begin their careers as pharmacists, the quality of healthcare can be expected to improve.

This study did have some limitations. First, as pharmacy students only had two required readings, comprehensive EBM items were not included in the EBM workshop. For example, relative risk and hazard ratios were used in the literature, so the preceptor provided descriptions of these ratios. Furthermore, although interpreting mean differences is also important for EBM, this was not covered in the workshop. Secondly, we did not evaluate how effective the KJ method was in the EBM workshop. Positive results might be due to the preceptor lecture or KJ method effectiveness or both. We will need to evaluate which domain is more effective in the next study. Finally, as the EBM workshop was conducted during one day and the post-workshop questionnaire was administered immediately after its conclusion, the long-term effects of the workshop are unclear. A follow-up study might be necessary to determine any long-term effects.

In conclusion, the results of this study suggest that our EBM workshop significantly enhanced student awareness of the importance of reading the clinical literature regularly. Therefore, reading current clinical literature prior to graduation is an important part of education for pharmacy students in Japan. It is therefore expected that pharmacy students who participated in our EBM workshop will contribute to improvements in the quality of the pharmacy profession in the future.

3.1 Japanese pharmacy education for current pharmacists -Journal Club as a Method of Improving Medical Terminology and Critical Reading Skills: Outcome Verification in the Department of Pharmaceutical Sciences at Tohoku University Hospital-

3.2 Background

Journal clubs are popular instructive methods among pharmacy students and pharmacists in the USA. These are often assigned to APPE pharmacy students by their preceptors.(Arif *et al.*, 2012) Generally, the journal club is one of the methods to update current medical knowledge for pharmacists in the USA. It is an instructive group meeting in which attendees discuss current clinical literature critically and evaluate what is applicable to real clinical situations.(Kirchhoff and Beck, 1995) The advantage of this group meeting is that attendees are able to update new information regarding current pharmacotherapy and oral presenters and attendees can experience critical evaluation of clinical literature.(Kleinpell, 2002) If this method is adapted to pharmacy practice in Japan, Japanese pharmacists will be able to utilize high-evidence information from the clinical literature to daily practice.

3.3 Objectives

To improve pharmacy practices at a university hospital, a journal club advancement program was established and the pedagogical results examined with pharmacists who can critically read clinical literature.

3.4 Methods

3.4.1 Journal club advancement program

3.4.1.1 Preceptor trainings

Pharmacists who have greater than five years' experience were recruited as candidates to be preceptors in training. The preceptor-education program consisted of 16 components, done in one hour/week blocks. The first to seventh blocks emphasized medical terminology. A medical terminology book was required of preceptor candidates. Each block included an "Individual Readiness Assurance Test" (IRAT) and a "Group Readiness Assurance Test" (GRAT). Individual candidates answered IRAT questions regarding medical terminology; then all candidates reconfirmed answers with explanations on the GRAT. The IRAT and GRAT were the same test. In the eighth and ninth blocks, I gave lectures to preceptor candidates using the Avoiding Cardiovascular Events through Combination Therapy in Patients Living with Systolic Hypertension (ACCOMPLISH) trial(Jamerson *et al.*, 2008) to show how to critically read clinical literature. These steps were explained in a journal club guide with 50 questions on important points of how to critically read clinical literature that I translated into Japanese. After that, all candidates performed oral presentations in the 10th to 15th blocks. At this time, they selected current clinical literature published within six months and created a two-page handout. The handout consisted of 11 items, namely "background," "purpose," "methods," "patients," "treatment," "outcome," "statistics," "results," "critique" (advantages and disadvantages), "conclusions," and "recommendations." In the 13th to 15th blocks, I evaluated oral presentations by candidates using an evaluation sheet. Finally, in the 16th block, the KJ method (Scupin, 1997) was performed with all candidates to discuss preparedness as preceptors. Candidates discussed the topic of "important things as journal club preceptors" in a small group (Table 2).

3.4.1.2 General participants' trainings

Trained preceptor candidates became real preceptors after finishing the journal club advancement program. Each of them educated two pharmacists as general participants. A schedule of this program did not include in the last block. The relationship between the preceptor trainings and the general participants' trainings was shown in Figure 16.

3.4.2 Medical terminology tests and questionnaires

Outcome verification of the journal club advancement program was performed with pre- and post- medical terminology tests (50 questions) and pre-and post-questionnaires (seven-point Likert scale). Pre- and post- medical terminology tests were the same. Pre-and post-questionnaires were shown in Figure 17A and 17B, respectively.

3.4.3 Statistical analysis

Paired t-tests were performed to compare pre-medical terminology with post-medical terminology tests. Wilcoxon signed rank test was performed to compare pre- and post-questionnaires. P values less than 0.05 indicated statistical significance.

3.4.4 Ethical considerations

The ethics committee of Tohoku University School of Medicine approved this study. At the beginning of the study, oral and written explanations were provided. Participation in the medical terminology tests and questionnaire surveys indicated provision of informed consent.

3.5 Results

Seven preceptor candidates participated in the journal club advancement program. I educated three and four candidates in the first and second term, respectively. Eleven general participants participated in the program and each preceptor educated two participants.

Fourteen pharmacists (78%) responded that they had read English or Japanese clinical literature. Sixteen pharmacists (89%) responded they had never learned how to critically read clinical literature (Figure 18). Medical terminology tests for preceptor candidates showed that scores increased from 34.7 ± 3.5 (average $\pm$ SE) to 45.3 ± 1.4 (P = 0.007; Table 3). Pharmacists' responses to "AT THIS TIME, do you think that pharmacists at hospitals need to habitually read clinical literature?" were 5.3 ± 0.8 and 6.4 ± 0.4 on pre- and post-questionnaires, respectively (P = 0.125). Pharmacists' responses to "AT THIS TIME, are you confident in reading clinical literature?" significantly increased from 2.0 ± 0.4 to 4.6 ± 0.3 (P = 0.008). Pharmacists' responses to "AT THIS TIME, can you discuss the results of clinical literature with physicians and nurses?" significantly increased from 1.9 ± 0.4 to 4.4 ± 0.4 (P = 0.008). Pharmacists' responses to "AT THIS TIME, do you habitually read clinical literature?" significantly increased from 1.4 ± 0.3 to 4.4 ± 0.2 (P = 0.008; Table 4).

Medical terminology tests for general participants showed that scores increased from 32.9 ± 2.0 to 44.5 ± 1.4 (P = 0.0004; Table 3). General participants' responses to "AT THIS TIME, do you think that pharmacists at hospitals need to habitually read clinical literature?" were 5.9 ± 0.4 and 6.3 ± 0.2 on pre- and post-questionnaires, respectively (P = 0.375). General participants' responses to "AT THIS TIME, are you confident of reading clinical literature?" significantly increased from 1.4 ± 0.2 to 4.0 ± 0.4 (P = 0.004). General participants' responses to "AT THIS TIME, can you discuss the results of clinical literature with physicians and nurses?" significantly increased from 1.6 ± 0.3 to 4.2 ± 0.4 (P = 0.005). General participants' responses to "AT THIS TIME, do you habitually read clinical literature?" significantly increased from 2.0 ± 0.5 to 4.0 ± 0.5 (P = 0.008; Table 4).

Participants' impressions of the program's good and bad points are shown in Tables 5 and 6, respectively.

3.6 Discussion

To improve pharmacy practices in the pharmacy at Tohoku University Hospital, a journal club advancement program was established and its pedagogical results examined with pharmacists who can critically read clinical literature. As a result, both preceptor candidates and general participants learned medical terminology and were more confident of reading clinical literature, indicating that this program is useful to teach current pharmacists at a hospital to habitually read clinical literature.

Scores of both pre- and post-questionnaire were high and pharmacists in the program think that it is necessary to habitually read clinical literature (Table 4). Additionally, 78% of participants in the program have read clinical literature before in either English or Japanese (Figure 19). On the other hand, most participants seldom habitually read clinical literature in the pre-questionnaire, suggesting that although they understood the necessity of reading clinical literature, they did not apply new information from current

34

clinical literature to daily pharmacy practice. Since the program showed that participants are able to habitually read clinical literature, it is expected that they would apply new information from current clinical literature with not only package inserts but also that interview forms in pharmacy practice would increase.

Many pharmacists responded that they had never learned how to critically read clinical literature. The pre-questionnaire revealed that most participants were not confident of reading clinical literature and were not able to discuss it with physicians and nurses, perhaps because they do not initially learn how to critically read clinical literature. As conventional pharmacy education in Japan did not include lectures/exercises on how to critically read clinical literature, it did not help pharmacists who were not initially confident. Pharmacy students in the USA learn how to critically read clinical literature in classes on drug literature evaluation or drug information. (Burkiewicz and Komperda, 2009; Motl *et al.*, 2006) In addition, journal clubs are often assigned to APPE pharmacy students.(Arif *et al.*, 2012) In this situation, pharmacy students in the USA are able to critically evaluate current clinical literature prior to graduation. On the other hand, in Japan, the MCC was revised in 2015 and "critically reading clinical literature" was included in it to understand a basic concept of EBM. Henceforth, pharmacy students who received revised MCC will be able to critically evaluate clinical literature. However, the approach in this study is necessary for already practicing pharmacists and it is necessary to continue the approach.

One of the main characteristic points of the program is that it places emphasis on learning medical terminology in its first half. If participants who are not good at reading English try to understand clinical literature written in English at the beginning of the program, they are unlikely to continue because of the language barrier. Therefore, learning medical terminology was taught in the first half of the program to get used to English. Participants systematically learned meanings of prefixes and suffixes of medical terms and checked points of critically reading clinical literature in the second half of the program. Some participants noted that this program decreased the language barrier to some degree, suggesting that this program is useful for participants who do not understand

English well.

Previous reports in Japan introduced some approaches to journal clubs. For example, a style of connecting multi facilities using Skype, a journal club in occupational therapy education, a journal club held in a pharmacy at a university hospital, and so on were reported. However, these reports did not evaluate the effectiveness of the approaches. The approach in the pharmacy at Tohoku University Hospital was an instructive method for current pharmacists in the pharmacy at the present time; skills of critically reading clinical literature are necessary for not only pharmacists at university hospitals but also those at community hospitals and pharmacies. If expanding the approach to community areas is considered, the journal club with Skype would be applicable.

This study did have some limitations. The program consisted of 16 blocks and was held one hour/week. However, because of participants' business, the program was not in fact held every week. Actually, it took about six months for completion. Since the program adopted a small group style of 2–3 participants per group, numbers were limited. Nonetheless, as the program can certainly educate participants, it is necessary to steadily continue the program. Additionally, although all scales on the post-questionnaires significantly increased except for the question of necessity of reading clinical literature, scales stayed about four on a seven-point Likert scale, suggesting that the approach could be improved and that it is necessary for participants to develop more confidence. This approach mainly emphasized reading articles of large scale randomized clinical trials. Henceforth, the program will be revised to include how to interpret non-inferior trials and retrospective studies to lead to an enhanced program and increased confidence for participants.

Pharmacists who are not initially interested in reading clinical literature will be future problems for the journal clubs. The program adopted a small group style and a closed environment. Because of that, non-participant pharmacists in the pharmacy cannot know what kind of knowledge they would be able to obtain from the journal club. Therefore, journal club descriptions will be presented to all pharmacists in the pharmacy by oral presentations from the participants who finished the program. This will be a good opportunity to learn what knowledge and skills the participants obtained from the program. Additionally, in the USA, lack of interest in the journal club or few participants are problematic.(Stallings *et al.*, 2011) In order to improve these problems, selection of clinical literature which is applicable to the patients treated by participants and a debate discussion with two participant groups are proposed.(Stallings *et al.*, 2011) These hints will be considered to improve the journal clubs.

In conclusion, to improve pharmacy practices at Tohoku University Hospital, a journal club advancement program was established and the pedagogical results were examined with pharmacists who can critically read clinical literature. As a result, it is clear that the program is useful and that homogeneous educational effects are expected. This approach will be continued to improve pharmacy practices.

4. Summary

To clarify the problems of drug information education in Japan, a comparative survey of pharmacists' perceptions of clinical literature accessibility between Japan and the USA was performed. Japanese pharmacists did not sufficiently apply information from the clinical literature in practice because conventional pharmacy education in Japan did not give lectures/exercises to pharmacy students on how to critically read clinical literature. I thought that some approaches are necessary to fill the gap between Japan and the USA and created programs for pharmacy students and current pharmacists – the EBM workshop for students and the journal club advancement program for current pharmacists. It is clear that these two programs are useful instructive methods to enhance pharmacy students' awareness of the importance of reading clinical literature and to improve current pharmacists' skills in evaluating clinical literature, respectively. In particular, the journal club advancement program has expanded to the community in Miyagi prefecture. The journal club program for pharmacists at community hospitals in Miyagi prefecture began in 2014. I have taught them to critically read clinical literature. I hope that some of them will be journal club leaders at their hospital pharmacies in the future and the number of pharmacists who are able to evaluate clinical literature and apply information to real pharmacy practices will

increase. I will be glad if my approaches enhance the quality of

Japanese pharmacy practice in the future.

Arif S. A., Gim S., Nogid A., Shah B. (2012) Journal clubs during advanced pharmacy practice experiences to teach literature-evaluation skills. *Am J Pharm Educ,* **76**, 88.

Bookstaver P. B., Rudisill C. N., Bickley A. R., McAbee C., Miller A. D., Piro C. C., Schulz R. (2011) An evidence-based medicine elective course to improve student performance in advanced pharmacy practice experiences. *Am J Pharm Educ,* **75**, 9.

Burkiewicz J. S., Komperda K. E. (2009) An elective course on landmark trials to improve pharmacy students' literature evaluation and therapeutic application skills. *Am J Pharm Educ,* **73**, 31.

Cohn J. N., Tognoni G. (2001) A randomized trial of the angiotensin-receptor blocker valsartan in chronic heart failure. *N Engl J Med,* **345**, 1667-1675.

Ikeda N. R., Schwartz D. G. (1992) Impact of end-user search training on pharmacy students: a four-year follow-up study. *Bull Med Libr Assoc,* **80**, 124-130.

Jamerson K., Weber M. A., Bakris G. L., Dahlof B., Pitt B., Shi V., Hester A., Gupte J., Gatlin M., Velazquez E. J. (2008) Benazepril plus amlodipine or hydrochlorothiazide for hypertension in high-risk patients. *N Engl J Med,* **359**, 2417-2428.

Kirchhoff K. T., Beck S. L. (1995) Using the journal club as a component of the research utilization process. *Heart Lung,* **24**, 246-250.

Kleinpell R. M. (2002) Rediscovering the value of the journal club. *Am J Crit Care,* **11**, 412-414.

McMurray J. J., Ostergren J., Swedberg K., Granger C. B., Held P., Michelson E. L., Olofsson B., Yusuf S., Pfeffer M. A. (2003) Effects of candesartan in patients with chronic heart failure and reduced left-ventricular systolic function taking angiotensin-converting-enzyme inhibitors: the CHARM-Added trial. *Lancet,* **362**, 767-771.

Motl S. E., Timpe E. M., Eichner S. F. (2006) Evaluating the accuracy of health news publications in a drug literature evaluation course. *Am J Pharm Educ,* **70**, 83.

Phillips J. A., Gabay M. P., Ficzere C., Ward K. E. (2012) Curriculum and instructional methods for drug information, literature evaluation, and biostatistics: survey of US pharmacy schools. *Ann Pharmacother,* **46**, 793-801.

Scupin R. (1997) The KJ Method: A Technique for Analyzing Data Drived from Japanese Ethnology. *Hum. Org.,* **56**, 233-237.

Stallings A., Borja-Hart N., Fass J. (2011) New Practitioners Forum: Strategies for reinventing journal club. *Am J Health Syst Pharm,* **68**, 14-16.

Timpe E. M., Motl S. E., Eichner S. F. (2006) Weekly active-learning activities in a drug information and literature evaluation course. *Am J Pharm Educ,* **70**, 52.

Wang F., Troutman W. G., Seo T., Peak A., Rosenberg J. M. (2006) Drug information education in doctor of pharmacy programs. *Am J Pharm Educ,* **70**, 51.

Publication

"Effects of an Evidence-Based Medicine Workshop on Japanese Pharmacy Students' Awareness Regarding the Importance of Reading Current Clinical Literature" was originally published in the *Journal of Pharmaceutical Health Care and Sciences* 2015 1:23.

Figure 1 A questionnaire to pharmacists in Florida

Figure 2 Background of pharmacists in Miyagi and Florida

Figure 3 Habitually reading clinical literature

Figure 4 Necessity of reading clinical literature

Figure 5 Pharmacists who habitually read clinical literature

Figure 6 Reasons why pharmacists did not habitually read clinical literature

Figure 7 How to critically read clinical literature

("Have you ever read English or Japanese clinical literature?" and "Have you ever learned how to critically read clinical literature before?" n=18)

Table 1 Results of the pre- and post-workshop questionnaires on EBM (n=37).

EBM: Evidence-based medicine. Data are expressed as mean ± standard error (SE).

Table 2 Schedule of preceptor trainings

Table 3 Results of medical terminology test

Table 4 Results of questionnaires (candidates of preceptor: n=7, general participants: n=11)

Table 5 Results of questionnaires ("Please tell us good points of the program")

Table 6 Results of questionnaires ("Please tell us bad points which should be improved")

Figure 1

Pharmacist Perception of Clinical Literature Accessibility Survey
Comparisons of Japan and USA

INSTRUCTIONS: Please either check or fill in the appropriate blanks. Submit your survey online. Even if you do not work in a pharmacy currently, we still ask you to complete the survey. Please answer the questions the best you can.

SECTION 1: INFORMATION ABOUT YOURSELF

1. Please check the one item that best describes your primary place of employment.
   ___ Hospital pharmacy
   ___ Community pharmacy
   ___ Others _____

2. If you are a hospital pharmacist, which of the following best describes your current position?
   ___ Clinic-based pharmacist
   ___ Staff pharmacist
   ___ Others _____

3. How long have you been a pharmacist since obtaining your pharmacist license?
   ___ 1-5 years
   ___ 6-10 years
   ___ 11-15 years
   ___ 16-20 years
   ___ 21-25 years
   ___ 26-30 years
   ___ More than 30 years _____

SECTION 2:   PHARMACY RELATED CLINICAL LITERATURE

4. Please response the question SUBJECTIVELY. Do you HABITUALLY read pharmacy related clinical literature?
   1. Yes (Go to Q5 and Q6)   2. No (Go to Q7)

5. On average, how often do you read clinical literature every month?
   ___ Less than once every month
   ___ Once every month
   ___ Twice every month
   ___ Three times every month
   ___ Four times every month
   ___ Five times every month

Figure 1

___ More than 5 times every month _____

6. Why do you HABITUALLY read clinical literature?
   ___ Necessary in practice
   ___ For myself education
   ___ Other _____

7. What is the main reason that you do NOT habitually read clinical literature?
   ___ I have no necessity to read clinical literature
   ___ I have no time to read clinical literature
   ___ I do not have access to clinical literature
   ___ Economic issues
   ___ Language barrier
   ___ Other _____

8. Do you think that the pharmacist needs to read clinical literature as part of his/her regular professional obligations?
   1. Yes   2. No

9. Please rate your <u>ability</u> to critique/analyze clinical literature.
   Accept it as written/Do not critique   Thoroughly Critique/Analyze
                          1   2   3   4   5   6   7

10. To what extent did you learn how to critically read clinical literature when you were a student-pharmacist?
   Not at all   1   2   3   4   5   6   7   Yes

11. To what extent do you apply the information you obtain from clinical literature to your daily responsibilities?
   Rarely/Never   1   2   3   4   5   6   7   Frequently

12. Do you have access to any clinical studies in your current work environment?
   Not at all   1   2   3   4   5   6   7   Yes, I have easy access.

13. Do you serve as a "preceptor" for student pharmacists?
   ___ Yes (Go to Q14)
   ___ No

14. As a preceptor, do you give your student-pharmacists clinical literature reading assignments?
   1. Yes   2. No

THANK YOU VERY MUCH FOR YOUR HELP!

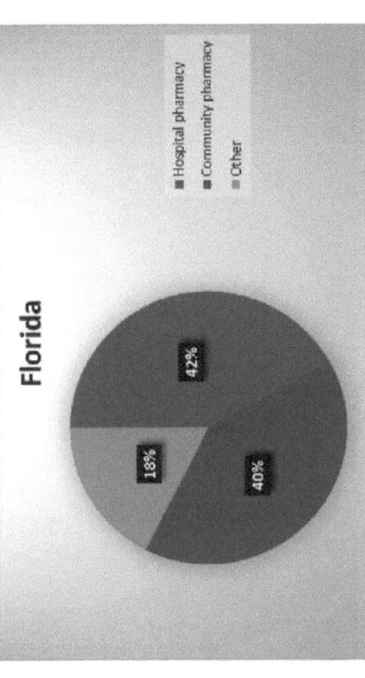

Miyagi

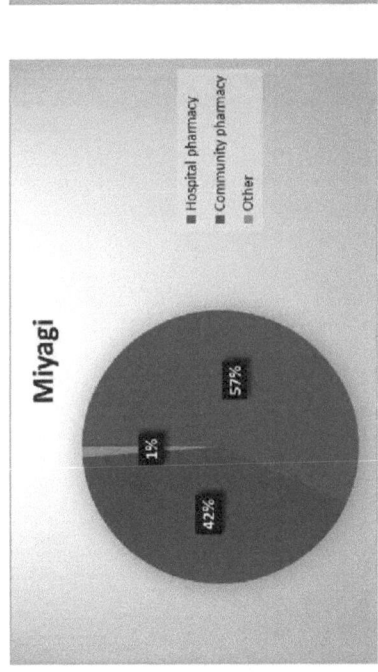

Florida

Miyagi n=605
Florida n=171

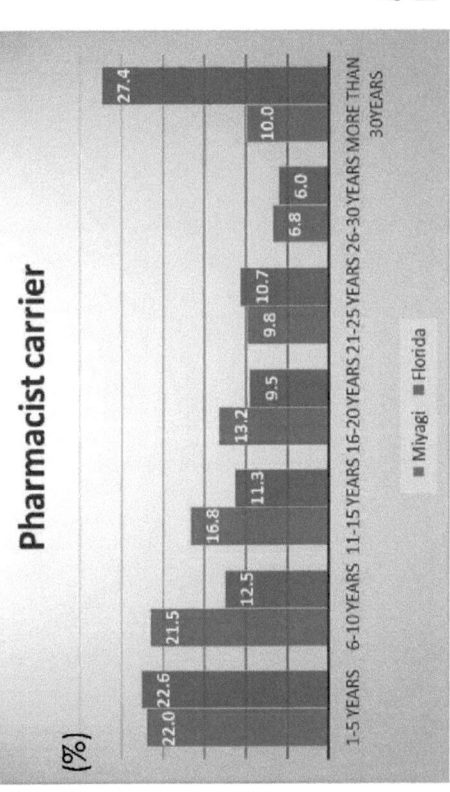

Miyagi n=591
Florida n=168

Figure 2

Do you HABITUALLY read pharmacy related clinical literature?

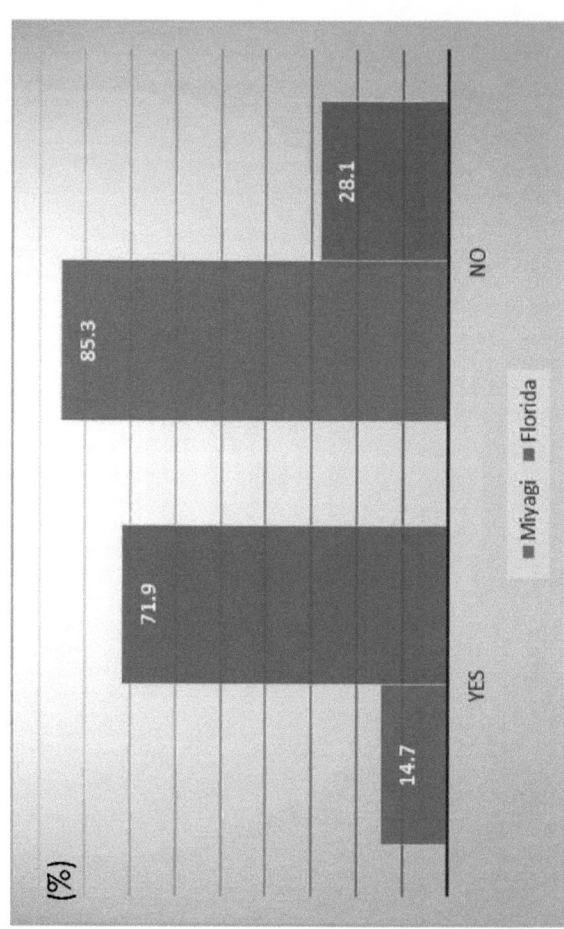

Miyagi n=597
Florida n=167

Figure 3

Do you think that the pharmacist needs to read clinical literature as part of his/her regular professional obligations?

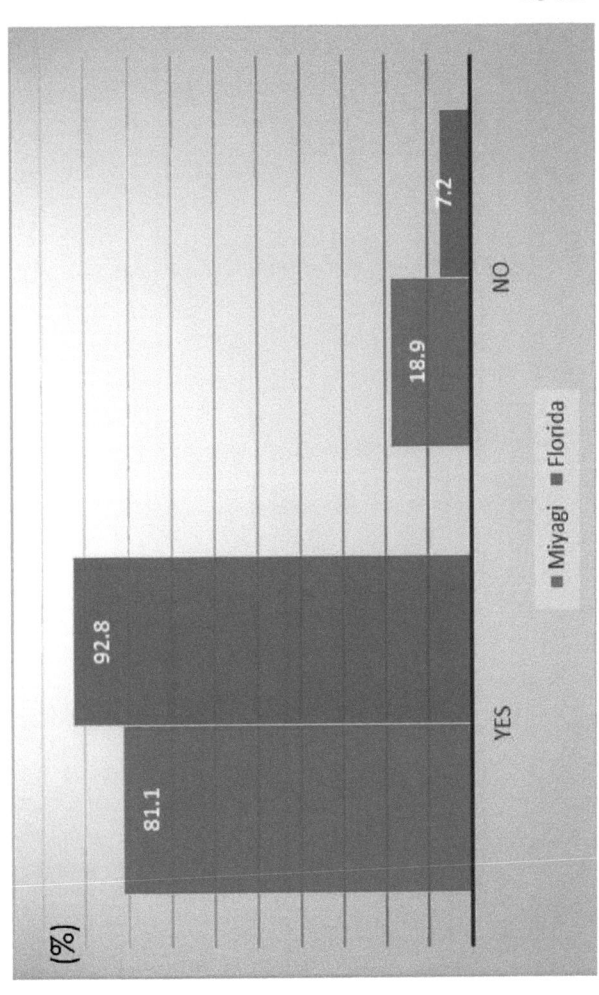

Miyagi n=594
Florida n=167

Figure 4

How often do you read clinical literature every month?

Miyagi n=85
Florida n=117

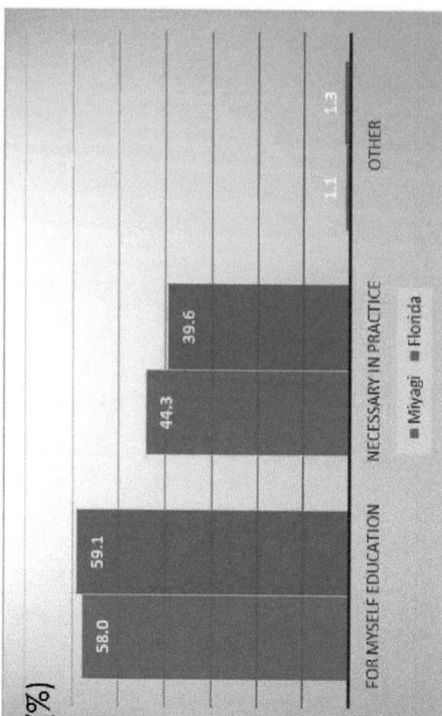

Why do you HABITUALLY read clinical literature?

Miyagi n=91
Florida n=159

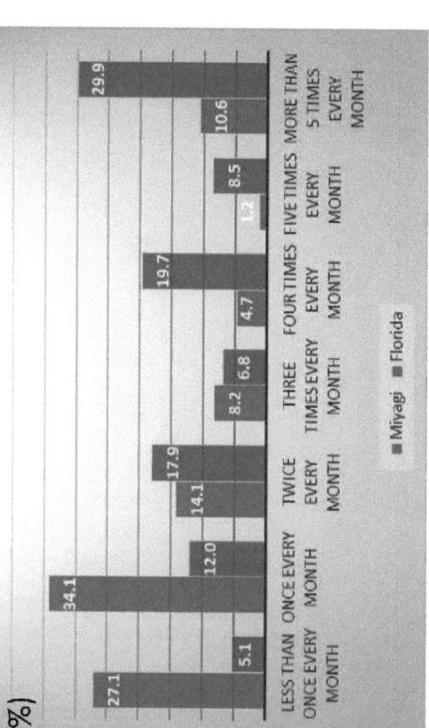

Figure 5

What is the main reason that you do NOT habitually read clinical literature?

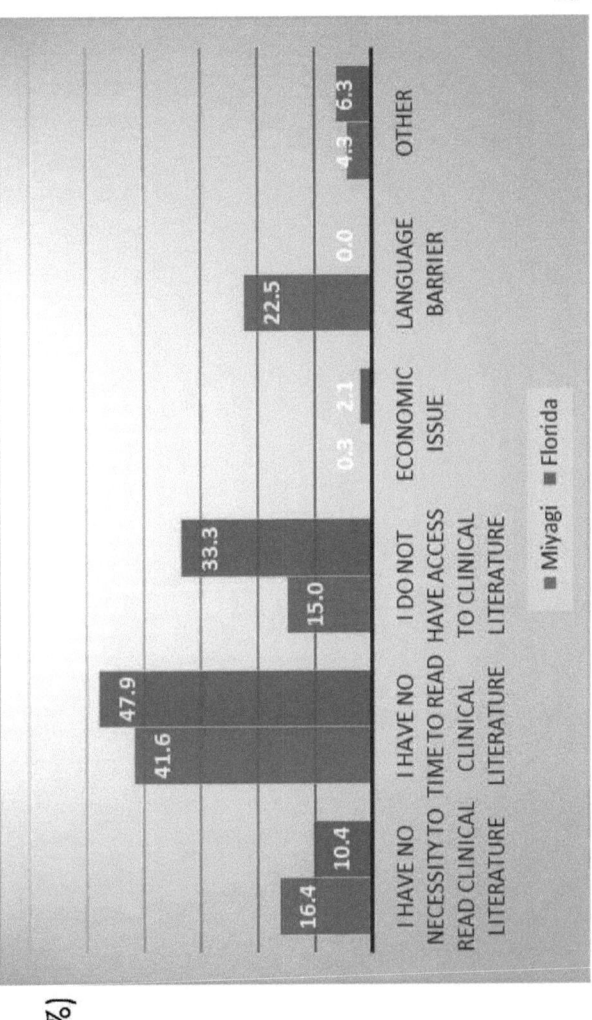

Miyagi n=654
Florida n=48

Figure 6

Rate your ability to critique/analyze
clinical literature

Miyagi n=591
Florida n=168

To what extent did you learn how to
critically read clinical literature when you
were a student-pharmacist?

Miyagi n=590
Florida n=170

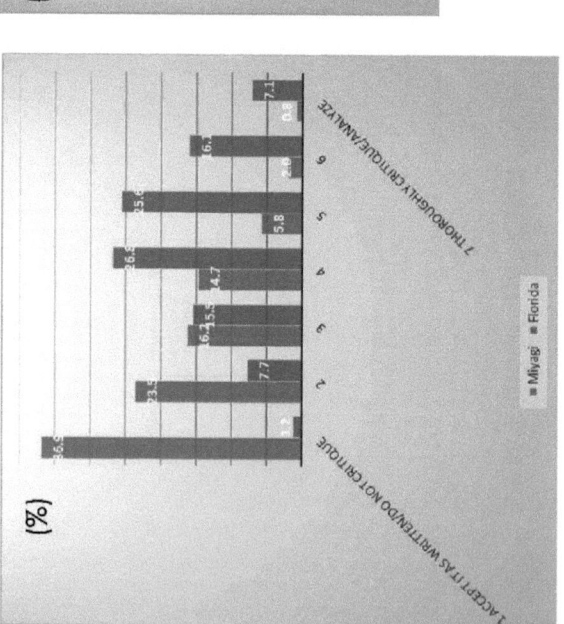

Figure 7

To what extent do you apply the information you obtain from clinical literature to your daily responsibilities?

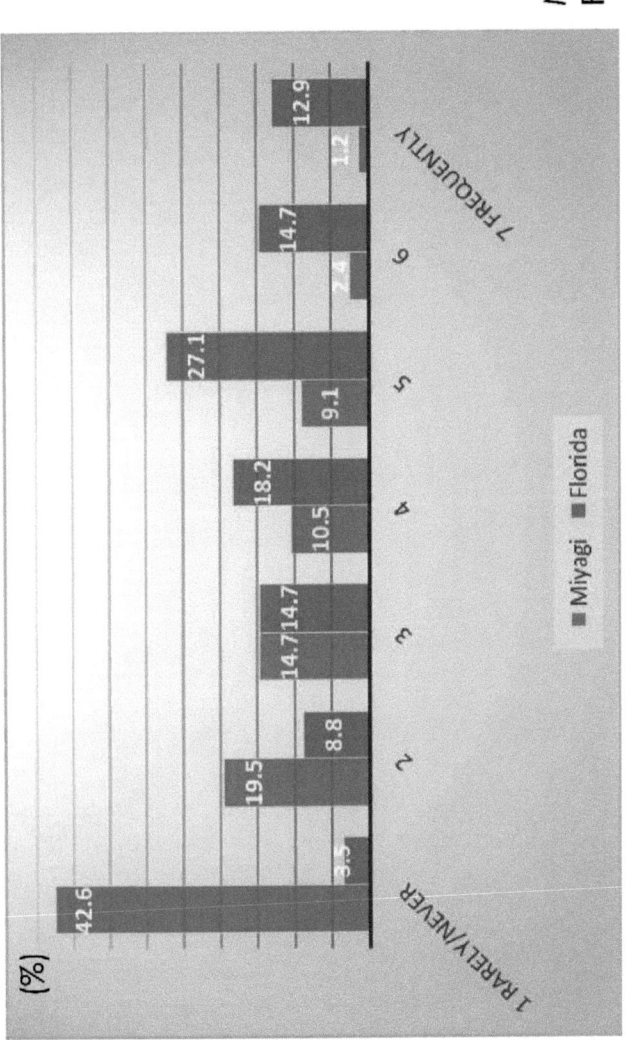

Miyagi n=573
Florida n=170

Figure 8

Do you have access to any clinical studies in your current work environment?

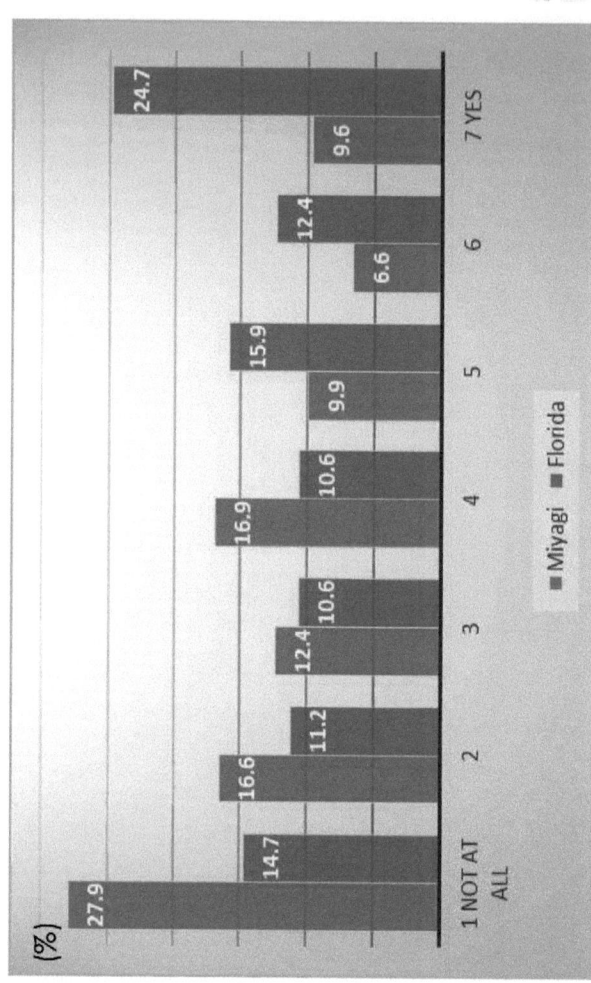

Figure 9

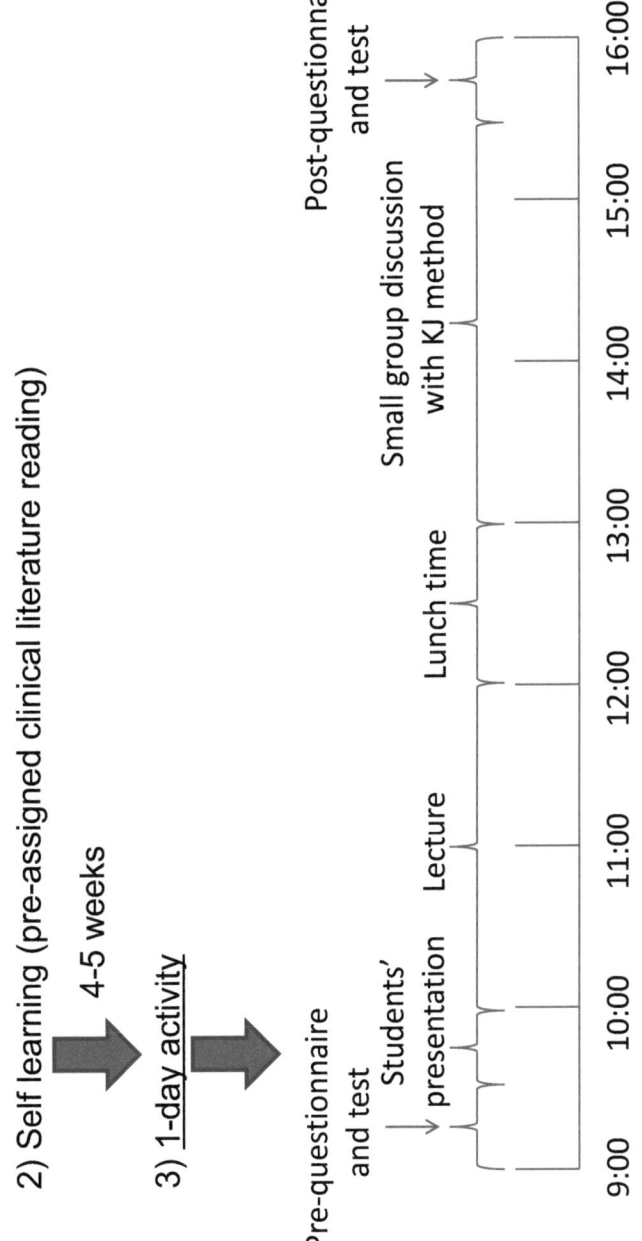

1) Orientation (2 required readings and 1 therapeutic guideline)

2) Self learning (pre-assigned clinical literature reading)

4-5 weeks

3) 1-day activity

Pre-questionnaire and test

Students' presentation

Lecture

Lunch time

Small group discussion with KJ method

Post-questionnaire and test

9:00   10:00   11:00   12:00   13:00   14:00   15:00   16:00

Figure 10

Cardiologist: "I think the symptoms of the patient with heart failure in room #905 have been gradually worsening. Standard treatment was performed. Adding an angiotensin receptor blocker (ARB) is a good option for her. Excuse me, pharmacist, could you please tell me which ARB is recommended for heart failure? "

Pharmacist: "To confirm, she has been taking enalapril, right? Are you thinking about combination angiotensin-converting enzyme inhibitor (ACEI) and ARB therapy? I will check with the Drug Information (DI) pharmacist and let you know soon. "

Cardiologist: "Yes, thank you."

On the telephone

Pharmacist: "That's the question. Let me know as soon as you can."

DI pharmacist: "OK. I will do a literature search. Give me a little time."

Pharmacist: "All right. Thank you."

In the DI room

DI pharmacist: Combination ACEI and ARB therapy is discussed in a therapeutic guideline for patients with heart failure. Which ARB is better? Valsartan or candesartan?

Patient Information

55-year-old female
Chief complaint: shortness of breath
Prior medical history: diabetes, congestive heart failure (New York Heart Association functional classification III)
Examination: left ventricular ejection fraction (LVEF): 40% (2 months ago), 35% (3 days ago)
Medication:
Glimepiride (1 mg): 1 tab daily after breakfast
Enalapril (5 mg): 2 tabs daily after breakfast
Carvedilol (10 mg): 1 tab twice a day
Furosemide (40 mg): 1 tab twice a day after breakfast and lunch
Spironolactone (25 mg): 2 tabs twice a day after breakfast and lunch
Digoxin (0.125 mg): 2 tabs daily after breakfast
Tobacco and alcohol use: tobacco (-), alcohol (+)

Figure 11.

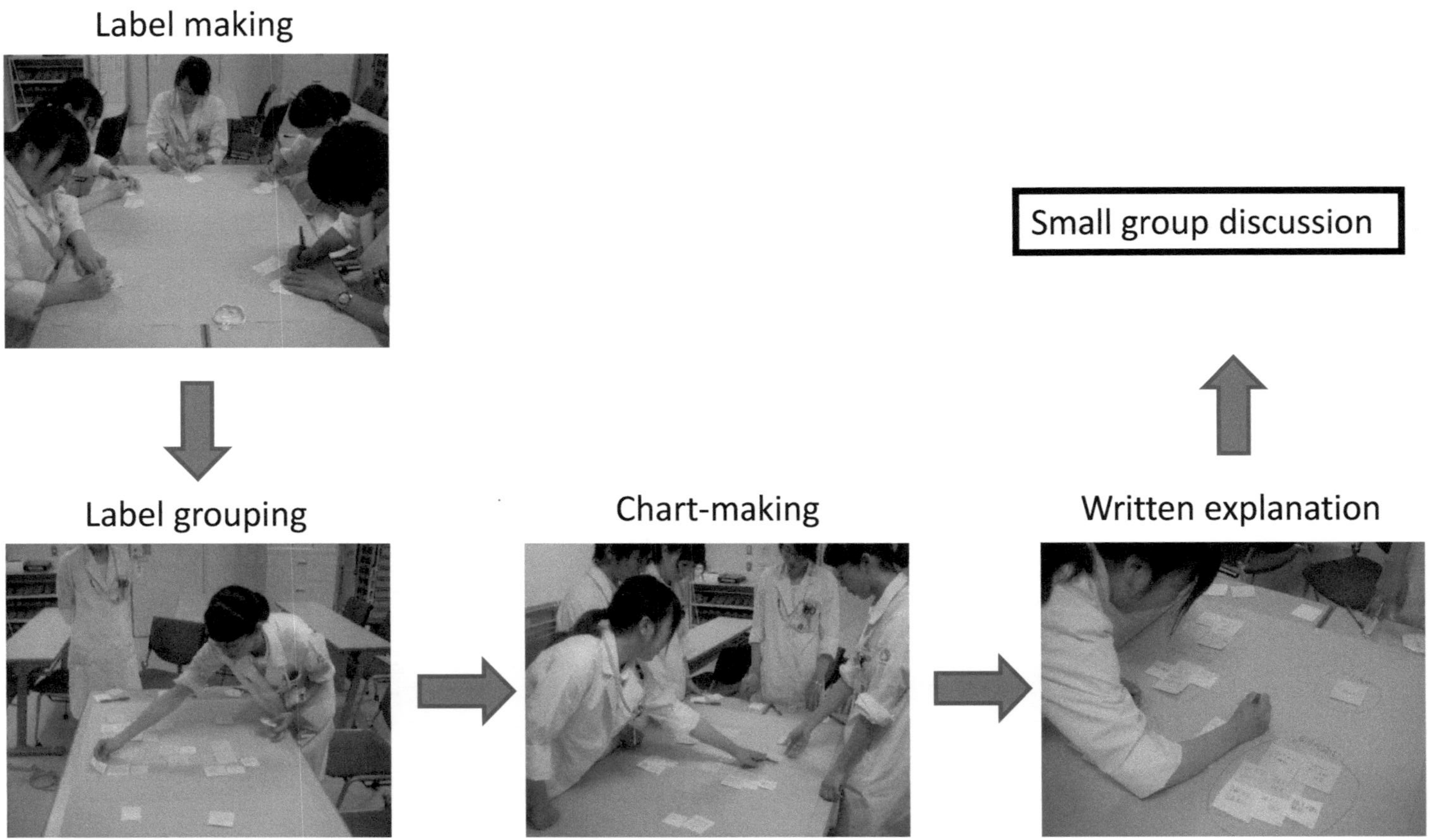

Label making

Label grouping

Chart-making

Written explanation

Small group discussion

Figure 12

Please circle the appropriate answer (Yes or No):

Q1. Have you ever read English or Japanese clinical literature?

                      Yes   No

Q2. Have you ever learned how to critically read clinical literature? (If Yes, proceed to Q3.)

                      Yes   No

Q3. How did you learn to critically read clinical literature?

(Please circle the most appropriate answer. If "Other", please specify.)

      A university lecture

      A pharmacy pre-lecture

      Self-learning

      A laboratory seminar

      A community lecture

      An academic meeting

      Other (   )

Please circle the number that best describes your view on each statement:

Q4. Pharmacists should read clinical literature regularly.

      Strongly disagree   Strongly agree

            1   2   3   4   5   6   7

Q5. I am confident in my ability to read clinical literature.

      Strongly disagree   Strongly agree

            1   2   3   4   5   6   7

Q6. If I were a hospital pharmacist, I could discuss treatment with nurses and physicians based on the results of clinical literature.

      Strongly disagree   Strongly agree

            1   2   3   4   5   6   7

Figure 13A

Please circle the number that best describes your view on each statement:

Q4. Pharmacists should read clinical literature regularly.

Strongly disagree   Strongly agree

1   2   3   4   5   6   7

Q5. I am confident in my ability to read clinical literature.

Strongly disagree   Strongly agree

1   2   3   4   5   6   7

Q6. If I were a hospital pharmacist, I could discuss treatment with nurses and physicians based on the results of clinical literature.

Strongly disagree   Strongly agree

1   2   3   4   5   6   7

Q7. What was the best thing about the EBM workshop?

Q8. What was the worst thing about the EBM workshop?

Q9. Please provide any additional comments here.

Figure 13B

Drug Information pharmacy experience   EBM test

Q1. EBM means "evidence based medicine".

     True   False

Q2. We are required to apply the principles of EBM when evaluating drug information.

     True   False

Q3. Randomized comparative studies are able to eliminate bias and minimize confounding factors.

     True   False

Q4. Typical types of observational studies include case-control studies and cohort studies.

     True   False

Q5. A randomized comparative study in clinical trials is a type of interventional study.

     True   False

Q6. An advantage of cohort studies over other types of studies that the cohort study tends to take less time and effort.

     True   False

Q7. Generally, a case-control study is called a prospective study.

     True   False

Q8. "Meta-analysis" describes when several independent studies are unified and evaluated statistically.

     True   False

Q9. "End-point" describes the meaning of treatment.

     True   False

Q10. "Surrogate end-point" is a concise end-point, essential in clinical study.

     True   False

Q11. Relative risk is a ratio of the patient with specific disease compared to the population exposed to a risk factor for that disease.

     True   False

Fig. 14

Q12. A relative risk of 1.0 is relatively high.   I.e., the percentage of individuals effected is high in risk factor-exposed group in comparison with risk factor-non-exposed group.

      True   False

Q13. The smaller the Number Needed to Treat (NNT) is, the more effective the treatment is.

      True   False

Q14. A meta-analysis was performed to evaluate the prophylactic effect of angiotensin converting enzyme inhibitors (ACEIs) for cardiovascular death in patients with acute myocardial infarction. The resulting odds ratio was 0.82 (95%CI 0.69-0.97) in comparison with the placebo group. Circle correct two answers.

1. There is no significant difference between the two groups because the odds ratio is close to 1.
2. ACEIs tend to decrease cardiovascular death because odds ratio is less than 1.
3. ACEIs do not decrease cardiovascular death significantly because a width of 95% confidential interval is 0.28.
4. The meta-analysis gives significant result because 95%CI does not exceed 1

Q15. Line up the following clinical trials in order, from the highest level of evidence to the lowest level of evidence. Circle the correct order below.
A. cohort study
B. randomized comparative study
C. meta-analysis of randomized comparative studies
D. case-control study

    1. A>C>B>D
    2. B>C>D>A
    3. B>A>D>C
    4. C>A>B>D
    5. C>B>A>D
    6. D>C>B>A

Fig.14 (continued)

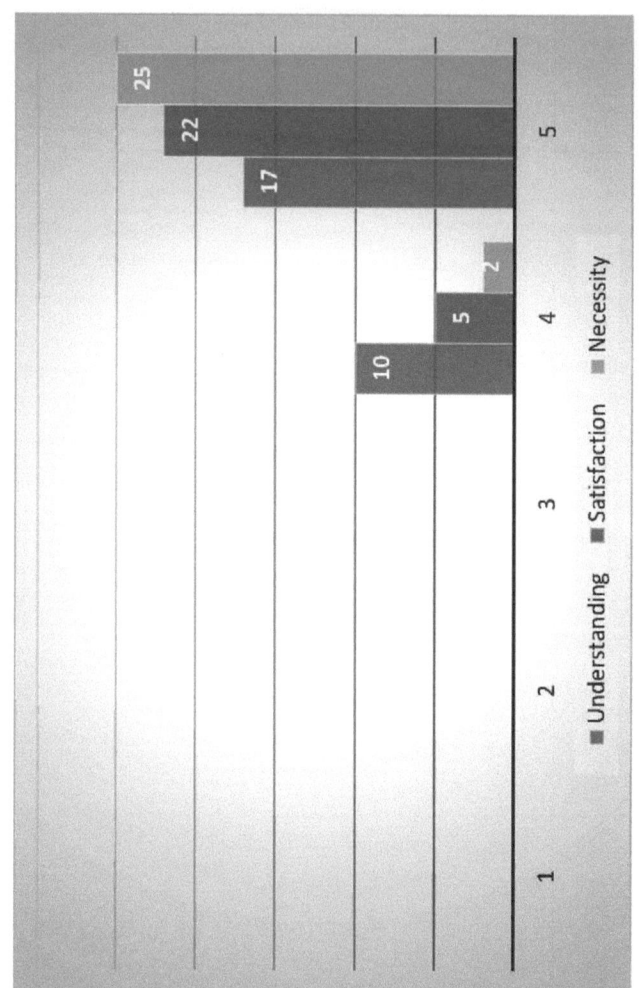

Figure 15

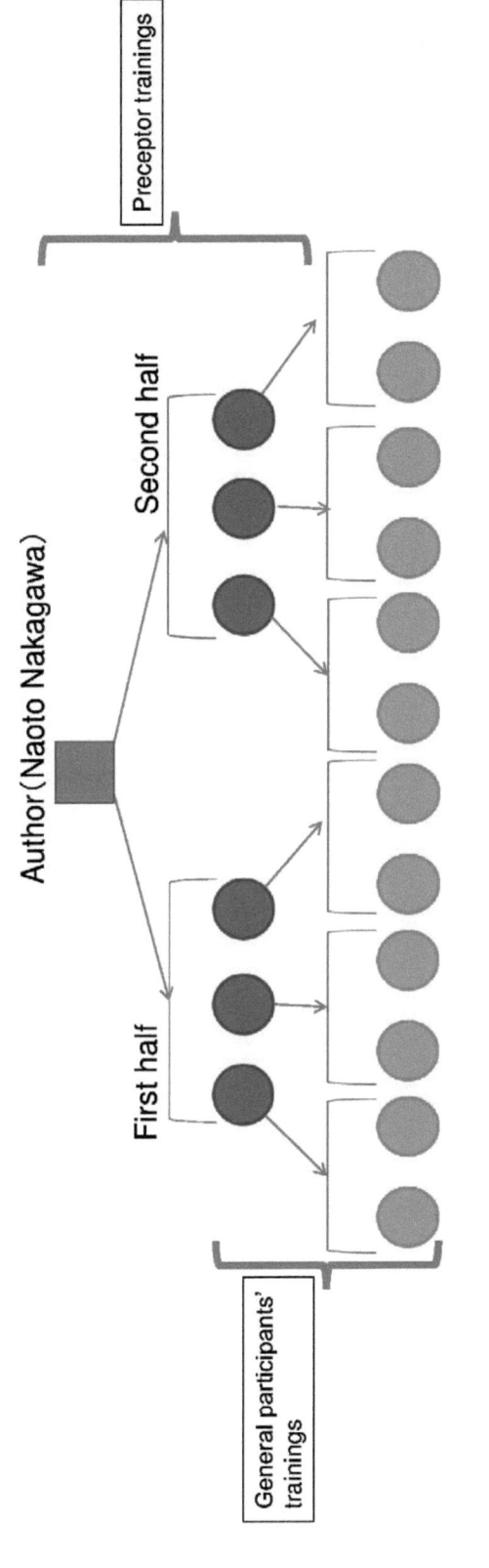

Figure 16

Table 1.

Question	Yes (%)	No (%)	Pre-	Post-	p value
Q1. Have you ever read English or Japanese clinical literature?	21 (57%)	16 (43%)			
Q2. Have you ever learned how to critically read clinical literature?	7 (19%)	30 (81%)			
Q3. How did you learn to critically read clinical literature?	University lecture: 6 Laboratory seminar: 1				
Q4. Do you think that pharmacists should read clinical literature regularly?			5.70±0.17	6.51±0.13	<0.0001
Q5. Are you confident in your ability to read clinical literature?			1.81±0.15	3.92±0.18	<0.0001
Q6. If you were a hospital pharmacist, could you discuss treatment with nurses and physicians based on the results of clinical literature?			2.49±0.22	3.86±0.21	<0.0001
EBM test (15 questions)			11.4±0.29	12.6±0.22	<0.0001

Table 2

Blocks	Contents	Note
—	Stocktaking of candidates of preceptor	Pre-medical terminology test, Pre-questionnaire
1	Medical terminology test 1 (IRAT and GRAT)	IRAT was returned to participants and GRAT was recovered
2	Medical terminology test 2 (IRAT and GRAT)	ditto
3	Medical terminology test 3 (IRAT and GRAT)	ditto
4	Medical terminology test 4 (IRAT and GRAT)	ditto
5	Medical terminology test 5 (IRAT and GRAT)	ditto
6	Medical terminology test 6 (IRAT and GRAT)	ditto
7	Medical terminology test 7 (IRAT and GRAT)	ditto
8	Journal club guide 1 with ACCOMPLISH trial	Lecture by author (Naoto Nakagawa)
9	Journal club guide 2 with ACCOMPLISH trial	ditto
10	Oral presentation by pharmacist A	
11	Oral presentation by pharmacist B	
12	Oral presentation by pharmacist C	
13	Oral presentation by pharmacist A	Achievement evaluation
14	Oral presentation by pharmacist B	ditto
15	Oral presentation by pharmacist C	ditto
16	KJ method "What are important things as preceptors of the journal club?"	Post-medical terminology test and post-questionnaire

*IRAT; Individual Readiness Assurance Test

GRAT; Group Readiness Assurance Test

Table 3

Medical terminology test (50 questions)	Pre	Post	P value
Candidates of preceptor (n=7)	34.7±3.5	45.3±1.4	0.007
General participants (n=11)	32.9±2.0	44.5±1.4	0.0004

Table 4

Questions	Subjects	Pre	Post	P value
"AT THIS TIME, do you think that pharmacists at hospitals need to habitually read clinical literature?"	Candidates of preceptor	5.3±0.8	6.4±0.4	0.125
	General participants	5.9±0.4	6.3±0.2	0.375
"AT THIS TIME, are you confident of reading clinical literature?"	Candidates of preceptor	2.0±0.4	4.6±0.3	0.008
	General participants	1.4±0.2	4.0±0.4	0.004
"AT THIS TIME, can you discuss with physicians and nurses based on the results of clinical literature?"	Candidates of preceptor	1.9±0.4	4.4±0.4	0.008
	General participants	1.6±0.3	4.2±0.4	0.005
"AT THIS TIME, do you habitually read clinical literature?"	Candidates of preceptor	1.4±0.3	4.4±0.2	0.016
	General participants	2.0±0.5	4.0±0.5	0.008

Table 5

"Please tell us good points of the program"
· I got some viewpoints of reading clinical literature
· I can habitually read clinical literature
· This program decreases the language barrier to some degree
· We can be friends who have same ambition
· We can share information regarding current clinical literature
· I can level up step by step
· My reading speed is increased
· I can consider by myself to apply information from current clinical literature to real clinical situation and increase my ability to evaluate clinical literature

Table 6

"Please tell us bad points which should be improved"
· It would take shorter time in the first half of the program and it would take more much time to read and evaluate clinical literature.   · Numbers of oral presentations by participants would be increased.   · The program needs how to do literature search and introduction of academic journals which have high impact factors.   · The program needs the block of understanding statistics.

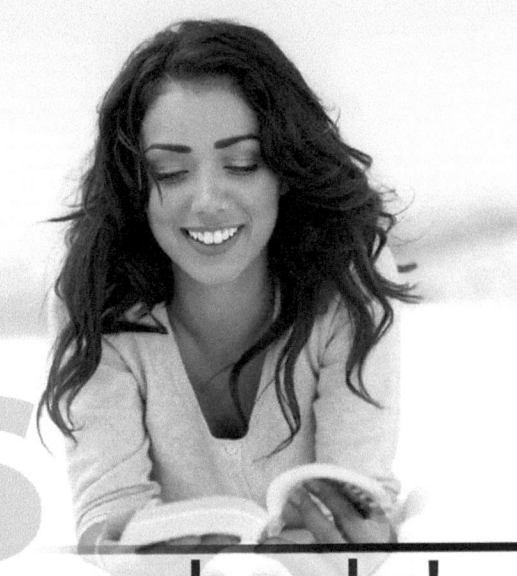
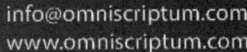
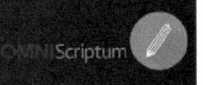

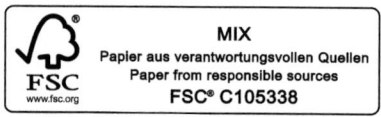
Printed by Books on Demand GmbH, Norderstedt / Germany